lose and maintain your weight
less or no colds
get rid of dandruff
get rid of psoriasis
free yourself of headaches
reduce or get rid of high blood pressure
get rid of sinus problems
prevent osteoporosis
control or get rid of colon problems
control diabetes two
etc. etc. etc.
prevent, stop or control, all kinds of illnesses, diseases, and allergies

You're Not **SICK**, You're **CLOGGED**

Yoga Matt

Founder of YogaMattAcademy.com

authorHOUSE®

AuthorHouse™
1663 Liberty Drive
Bloomington, IN 47403
www.authorhouse.com
Phone: 1 (800) 839-8640

Published by AuthorHouse 02/22/2019

ISBN: 978-1-5462-5253-5 (sc)
ISBN: 978-1-5462-5252-8 (e)

Library of Congress Control Number: 2018952993

Print information available on the last page.

This book is printed on acid-free paper.

It's not just a question of how long you are going to live. It's not just your quantity of life that's important. It's also your quality of life.

Most people choose to live with poor health and lack of understanding of what life really is all about. That makes us sick, unhealthy and unhappy. People just don't understand and are not being taught. There is a saying that says "health is wealth; peace of mind is happiness." When one realizes that money and things cannot buy health, true health. When one realizes that money and things cannot really buy happiness, then maybe we'll take a better look at ourselves, inside and out.

There are three main categories for good health and happiness. One is proper diet. The next is proper exercise. The last area of health and healing is proper living. Each one on a short-term basis will stand on its own, but long-term the three will have to work together.

Why We Get Sick

What if I told you we get sick because our body is clogged with the so-called food we put into our body. We also have physical problems because we don't do a gentle exercise to make our body strong and flexible. It's as simple as that. People just aren't supposed to have all these health problems. Why is it that the medical profession has to make it so complicated? A person can't keep putting stuff into their body that the bodies not meant to have. We just keep shoveling that stuff in as if it doesn't make a difference, but it does! We're also assuming and being told that basically everybody has a defective body. We have to be sick, have physical problems, it's normal! Normal? Having health problems is normal??? Having back problems, neck problems, shoulder problems, hip problems, knee problems, is normal? Osteoporosis is normal? Colon problems such as Crohn's disease, diverticulitis, ulcerative colitis are normal? It's just not normal; it's not! Without any question, it's not normal! None of this is normal, none of it! People aren't supposed to get sick like this. I've never seen anything like it. Almost every ad that I see on television, on certain channels, is about medication. People are really sick, and are sicker than I've ever seen in my life! Not only do I see older people sick, young people are having major health issues too. Young people have diseases that I've never seen at their age or anywhere close to their age. You mean to tell me that everybody's body is defective? You mean to tell me that we have to be sick? That we have no choice! If the body is the greatest machine ever created, and it is, then there must be things that we can do to regain our health, and to keep our health.

I hope you can feel my frustration in that last paragraph. I see children sick one after the other. Teenagers already with major health issues. Adults standing in long lines at drug stores and pharmacies waiting, almost desperate for their medication. There is an epidemic of obesity. Outpatient surgeries galore. Most of this does not have to be! Let me go on. Antidepressants being taken almost like candy. Sleeping pills, because people can't get sleep. Stimulants, such as coffee, chocolate, and sodas, because people can't wake up. Alcohol to relax the body, addictive drugs to kill the pain. We take antacids to stop the burning in the digestive system. We take laxatives because were so constipated. Does anybody ever stop to think why we have these problems? As I'm writing this book I'm saying to myself, what a mess! Alzheimer's increasing at an alarming rate. People have allergies, asthma, diabetes, the flu, the so called common cold, heart disease, cancer, and the list goes on and on. I'm sure by now you get the picture, and what a picture it is. Makes one want to gag, but guess what, we do have a choice!

Hooray! We actually do have a choice! You are not walking around in a defective human body! You just don't have the tools, the answers. So let me explain the answers; the rules of the game. What you can do to feel better, to look better, to be happier, to be healthier. Instead of having an unhealthy body, you'll have a fabulous body; healthier and happier body. When you look in the mirror, you'll have a smile on your face and a song in your heart!

The Human Body, The Greatest Machine Ever Created

First of all let me say this, your body is extremely tough. It can take a lot of abuse. Don't worry about the abuse you gave your body because that's in the past. The body can handle it on a temporary basis, not forever, but you can do some pretty bad things to it before it finally says, I give up.

And even when the body says I give up, there are things you can do so the body changes its mind.

Of course, the first thing is not to abuse your body at all. To take care of it right from the get-go. But for most of us we haven't done that. So the human body has built into it many ways to bring it back to health. I call that healthy state being centered, in balance, or in harmony. That's why I call the human body the greatest machine ever created, it can heal itself. The body can come back to health, back to balance. That's amazing!

So let's talk about how in its simplest form, this machine works. Why we get sick, and how we get better.

A Cold Is Not A Cold!

Let me say that again!

A Cold Is Not A Cold!

Ya got it?

A Cold Is Not A Cold!

Let's go on. So if a cold is not a cold, what is it?

A so called cold, is really a CLEANSING

A Cold Is Not A Cold

There are two times a year when we generally can catch a so-called common cold. That's when most people get sick with a runny nose, fever, coughing and possibly the flu. Those two times a year are in the fall and in the spring. We're told to be very careful so that we don't catch a cold. We're told that it's in the air. To be careful of people in a room, or in a store. The cold is just floating around, and we can catch a cold because we walked through that area. We're told to stay away from people because they might give us a cold, or we might get the flu. And we say to ourselves, we should have stayed away from that person, or I wish I hadn't been near that person, or don't go near that person because they're sick, and were going to get sick, because they're sick. Makes one's dizzy just thinking about it. Oh brother!

The question is, is the above true? Did you catch a cold, or did something else really happen? If you said something else really happened, you are correct. You didn't catch a cold. You shouldn't be upset with that person. You should be grateful that you were able to get what you got from that person. In fact go up to that person and say, thank you! What happened was instead of getting a cold they triggered in you a cleansing. Woo, they did you a favor! They gave your body a signal, somehow to cleanse, to detoxify. The question is how come we're not being taught that. If the body doesn't cleanse we get sicker and sicker if we hold back these cleansings. If we stop them we eventually get very sick. How come were not being taught that. A so called cold is not a cold at all. It's a way for the body to detoxify; a way for the body to cleanse. If by now I haven't made you really stop and think, then I suggest that you read the above paragraph from the top of the page all over again. KEEP ON READING IF YOU GET IT.

This is so important; this is finally why we get a major disease.

The body has backed up, and backed up, and backed up for years, and we have not allowed the body to cleanse all the debris that it's been clinging on to. There is so much junk in the body that it can't get rid of it. As I've said before, most human beings just don't have defective bodies.

So why does everybody have to go through this cleansing process where we get fevers, profusely runny noses, and tearing eyes? Why do we have to go through this? The reason is that the body is on overload. There is so much junk in the body and it can't get rid of it through normal channels! The body is starting to suffocate. We don't have defective bodies were literally slowly destroying the wonderful body we have.

The body is not a defective machine. It is created to last a long time, strong and healthy.

So let's talk about these so-called common colds that we all believe we have to have, for many at least once a year, for the rest of our lives, and for some people much more than twice a year. Did you ever hear the phrase you are what you eat? Did you ever think the body could handle all those different types of so-called foods you put into it? Did you ever stop and think that the body was designed in a specific way? That proper food keeps the body healthy, and whatever the body can't use of that real or proper food it discards? It discards what it can't use in normal ways because there's not much of it. Real foods such as fruits, vegetables, grains, beans, nuts, seeds and a little bit of possibly healthy meat. (*Notice I have no dairy products there whatsoever. We'll discuss that later.*)

Think about this one:

We actually take better care of our car than we do of ourselves. A car can't run on contaminated gasoline, and a car's engine will eventually break down if we use low-quality oil. So we take very good care of our car. We put high-quality oil in the engine and we change the oil every so many thousands of miles. We have to keep the air filter clean otherwise the car doesn't run right. We have to use the right octane gasoline otherwise the car won't run right. If we don't take care of our car it won't last long at all, and we'll have problems with it. If we don't run the car and it just sits, it starts to fall apart too. Doesn't that sound just like the human body!

I have a better story. The dashboard on a car has all kinds of warning lights, right? When one light goes on, what do we do? We take the car in to the mechanic and get it fixed. Once it's fixed then the light is turned off, correct? When we get a headache, which is a warning light, what do we do? We take a pain pill and we feel that the light goes off. The problem is that we never solved the reason for the headache, we just turned the light off. We never fixed the source of the problem. Think about that one!

Take the word cold, as in I have a cold. Change it to the word cleansing, as in my body is cleansing. I hope that makes so much more sense to you.

Let me explain the cleansing. What we been told for most of our lives is that we caught a cold. In reality that's not true! One way to look at it is a negative, and the other way is a positive. So let's go with the positive. The positive being our body is discharging toxins. Our body is going through a cleansing. A very normal process so that the body can stay healthy, in balance.

As I'm writing this book it occurred to me, that the flu may actually be an extreme cleansing. Do not let your body get to this point. If you do get the flu it's important to somehow slow the extreme cleansing down. Go to a doctor and do what is necessary to get temporarily better. Once you are temporarily better take care of yourself, and let the body cleanse slowly. By taking care of yourself I mean a much better diet, and an exercise program that absolutely works. I promise you I will teach you how to do this. My guess is that eventually these colds, including the flu, will disappear. If we take care of our body, just like a car, we will run for a lot of miles. Many, many years of good, happy health.

By the way, I use the word extreme cleansing. Diarrhea is an extreme cleansing that also needs to be stopped, because of possible dehydration. What we're looking for is a slow, moderate cleansing. One that over time, gives you the good health you deserve.

The following explains the many ways that the body will cleanse. There's probably more! Keep reading on. I promise you I will help you to understand this and learn how to do this.

The human body has many ways to automatically cleanse itself easily:

1 – One way is through the pores; we sweat! Even when we don't sweat the pores are gently releasing stored energy. We are constantly getting rid of toxins through our pores. One of the best areas to get rid of toxins is under the arms; the armpits. Over time as we eat healthier, as our diet improves, the body odor under the arms will slowly almost totally disappear. Drink plenty of good, clean water.

2 – The second way to release toxins is by passing urine out of the body. That's another reason why it's so important to drink plenty of water.

3 – The third way of removing waste (toxins), is by having a good bowel movement. A good bowel movement should be had every day so that the body stays healthy. Again, drink plenty of good clean water. Eat foods with water in them, such as fresh fruits and vegetables.

4 – The nose and eyes also release toxins, normally very gently. Smile when you cry! Crying, just plain, releases a lot of negative energy. (Not only toxins will be released but negative feelings and emotions, also.) Drink plenty of good clean water. Tears are water with toxins in them.

5 – As we exhale the lungs release some water vapor, and a little bit of other gases, such as carbon dioxide, which to the human being is a toxic substance.

Read on!

6 – Another way the body cleanses is by running a fever. Fevers are a good thing as long as the fever doesn't get too high. If the fever gets too high, of course we need to bring it down. The purpose of a fever is to burn out toxins. Low fevers let us know there's something wrong with our body, but it's the burning out of toxins that helps the human body to heal.

7 – Sleep is a very important way for the body to detoxify. What I'm talking about is natural and refreshing sleep. Natural and refreshing sleep is normal for every human being to have, at any age! Natural and refreshing sleep means no sleep drugs, of any kind, as they dull the mind and add impurities to the body. I would think sleep drugs slow the bodily functions down as well, so we don't detoxify in a normal way.

The above points are the main ways for the body to cleanse gently. Let's go over each point in an expanded way, so that you can understand and change your life, to feel better, and to be happier.

Here we go!

Point one is that the body detoxifies through the pores, the skin; that's very important! Many parts of the world including the Indian cultures, use sweat lodges to detoxify the body. Sometimes, I think about how the Roman Empire used their hot baths. They seemed to be very important, possibly to cleanse the body. Today we have our saunas and steam rooms, in many cases, to probably do the same thing.

It's very important to remember to drink plenty of good clean water, every day! Most people are dehydrated. People drink caffeinated sodas, they drink coffee and tea with caffeine, but in reality these products literally dehydrate the body, because they are diuretics! Sooooo, people think their drinking enough water, but they're probably drinking too little and maybe in some cases go into the minus column with fluids. In many cases people are very dehydrated, so you have to make sure that you drink plenty of good clean water. Probably from 60 – 120 ounces of water a day even after you've had your caffeine drinks. Without proper hydration, in the body, it's very difficult for the body to cleanse; to stay healthy. *Remember caffeine drinks can put you into the minus column because they are diuretics.

I just had a disgusting thought. Visualize a plum that turns into a prune, shriveling up; what a picture. Is that what our cells look like if we're dehydrated? Oh boy! Remember, your body is approximately 65 percent to 70 percent water.

Oh boy again! The body is 65% to 70% water. Take a good look at yourself in the mirror. Are you running close to empty, or is your gas tank up to the level it should be.

Okay, we detoxify a lot through the pores. Makes sense to me! I hope, it makes sense to you. So let me ask you a question. Why do we seal off the pores under the arms? Under the arms happens to be one of the best places for the body to cleanse. That's probably why they're so much body odor, so much junk is trying to get out.

When I was a boy people used deodorants. They didn't seal the pores, they did stop the body odor. Before that people used perfumes, colognes, and baking soda to soak up the moisture, and to cover up the body odor. But then, big companies started to push antiperspirants. These companies made us feel as if the damp spot on the shirt, from sweating, was embarrassing. They made us feel that it was wrong to sweat! So we all went out and bought antiperspirants. The problem is antiperspirants hold back the release of toxins, waste from the body. Sometimes those pores will stay sealed even if we don't use more antiperspirants for two or three days, before the pores finally open. When the pores are sealed the body can't breathe under the arms, which again is one of the most important areas for the body to cleanse. The interesting thing is, the purer the diet, the less body odor we have. I've said before, it's the animal products that generally cause the body odor. When I say animal products I mean, chicken, cows, fish, pigs, and any other animal that doesn't want to give up its life. The animal is literally putrefying in your body, and that dead animal smells. The animal was killed, slaughtered and it's slowly doing the same thing to you. How about a big, oh boy, or a big, oh brother, or maybe just holy crap. Am I getting to you yet? Am I starting to make sense? Somewhere, I believe, I've read that people are tattooing the pores under the arms closed, never to breathe again. I don't even know what to say to that, except throw up my arms in disgust.

!oh brother!

what are we thinking?

Read on

Diseases don't happen just because. They happen because we do things that just don't make sense. Sometimes, I wonder why we don't teach these important things in school, but we don't.

Many women wear makeup. That makeup can clog the pores; it probably does. Again, the body can't breathe. At least buy natural makeup. Wear makeup as few hours as possible. If the skin can't breathe it's only common sense that eventually a person is going to get sick.

Think about suntan lotions and creams. They must seal the pores too. Along time ago people wanted to get out of the sun when it was extremely hot, they took their breaks, their siestas. Now when the sun is hottest people bake in the sun because they think they look wonderful. So they put on suntan lotion to prevent their skin from burning. I would think that suntan lotion seals the pores. Better to be in the sun early in the day or late in the afternoon. The other thing is not only do the pores get rid of toxins, but they also may absorb such toxic creams that we use on the body in order to stay healthy. What a joke! So you're damned if you do, and you're damned if you don't. Protect yourself from the sun with a large umbrella, big hat, or stay out of that hot sun altogether.

You have to get smart, you have to read a lot, and you have to listen a lot. Like I say so many times to people, you have to be smarter than the average bear. To me, when you think clearly, blocking the pores makes no sense. Pores of the skin are one of the major ways for the body to cleanse, detoxify, release stored negative energy, waste. The more that waste is held back, that energy is pushed and stuffed into the body, the sicker we will become, it's as simple as that.

Water is the vehicle for waste to come out of the body

I bet you didn't know this. Air-conditioning closes the pores and dehydrates the body, just like a frost free refrigerator removes moisture from inside the refrigerator. It's important to open the windows, to get plenty of fresh air and the beautiful sunlight. Spend time outside, just don't bake in the sun. Nature is a wonderful healer. Go on a picnic, take a beautiful walk, eat great food, be with your family and/or friends, and smile. Now you've got it all!

Remember
Drink More Water

Drink More Water

Drink More Water

<u>Dehydration is a major reason why people are sick</u>

Moisture in the air is very important. Home heating, in the wintertime, whether from a furnace or a fireplace dries out the body! Lips get dry and cracked. Hands get very dry, that's why we use moisturizers. Remember to drink more healthy clean water. Dry skin is a sign of being dehydrated, and so is possibly a dry mouth. If your heart skips you may be dehydrated, that's all!

Point two is that the body releases a lot of waste through the urine, which is another very good reason why it's important to drink a lot of water. Remember, I said water, not sodas, or juice, coffee, or caffeinated teas, because they really don't take the place of water. Some are diuretics and make you urinate more, so people are essentially dehydrated. Good healthy clean water, keeps the body good and healthy. It's as simple as that. Again, drinking water from 60 –120 ounces a day should allow the body to cleanse properly.

**Just a note: chocolate is high in caffeine and high in altered fat. It is not only an upper and a diuretic but will also help to clog up the body. Chocolates should be eaten sparingly.

Every method of cleansing, that the body has, requires enough water. The Grand Canyon they say was created by the Colorado River. It's the water that carried debris down the river, over time, that created the huge Grand Canyon. The same thing happens in our body. The water carries the stuff that doesn't belong there, the debris, out of the body. Water also carries excesses, such as salt, out of the body.

To make sure that you drink enough water every day, make a chart showing you just how much water you're drinking, and mark the ounces off. Another way is to buy, in the supermarket, a 50 ounce bottle of water, and fill it up twice a day. (Just do not over do it.)

(I would think that smaller children need to drink water at the lower end of the ounces a day. It's important to check with your pediatrician to find out.)

Read On

Point three talks about having a bowel movement. Having a bowel movement every day is essential to good health. Not just a bowel movement, a healthy bowel movement, otherwise you're essentially constipated.

The only way to do that, to have a good bowel movement, is to drink enough water and to have fresh fruits, vegetables, cooked beans and grains, all which have enough roughage, so that you can have a healthy, good bowel movement. You'll notice that this kind of food has water in it and roughage both. If you're eating something that's dry, such as popcorn or dry toast, please add some oil to it, otherwise it just won't pass through the system easily. Animal products are also constipating. Too much processed food in the diet, besides causing other health issues is also constipating. I would think too much salt in the diet, because it causes the body to contract, would also be constipating. Having a good bowel movement every day should prevent the major diseases that we are seeing today, such as colon cancer, and other diseases. Eating good food, drinking plenty of good water, and having a good bowel movement every day, gives us a chance. A much bigger chance to stay healthy. Just as a car would clog up if the exhaust system didn't work properly, we clog up also and it will make us sick.

(Saying the word bowel movement is embarrassing to many people. I'm sitting in my chair thinking to myself. That's embarrassing? That's embarrassing, but what people consider okay and talk about is all kinds of colon diseases, like it's nothing! People can talk about the colon being removed, like it's nothing!

It seems like it's easier to talk about cancer and heart disease than eating good clean healthy food, and drinking pure water. Does that make any sense? On top of that, we're now justifying people being obese, like it's okay! Obesity is not okay! People that are overweight get sick, very sick, and they die, in many cases, much younger! Being obese is not okay; being overweight is not okay. It creates all kinds of health issues. *Again, being constipated is eventually going to make a person sick. Do I hear another, oh brother!

Remember, you have to be smarter than the average bear. Take responsibility for your life. Don't give your power over to other people or companies.

Point four is about the nose and eyes releasing toxins. When a person drinks enough water, the eyes may tear, and definitely the nose sometimes will run, just by drinking plenty of water.

Of course, we all have heard the expression, laughter is the best medicine. Well, I will tell you, so is crying. When a person cries they release water, tears. In those tears is a lot of waste, a lot of negative stored energy. So when you cry, give yourself a pat on the back and try to keep the crying going. Don't let anybody tell you not to cry. The reason you feel better is because you have released a lot of energy, a lot of toxins. Crying and laughing can help somebody to feel much better, sometimes pretty darn fast.

**I do not believe that onions that cause eyes to tear, release toxins. Anything is possible.

Point five has to do with the lungs. By drinking a lot of water, by staying away from bad food, by deleting all dairy products out of your diet, or at least most, and by learning how to cleanse your lungs, which is a yoga exercise, many of the problems people are having with their lungs will probably disappear. People eating real food and learning how to cleanse their lungs, don't have the common problems today such as asthma. I have helped many people get off of their inhalators and either put their problems into remission, or get rid of their problems altogether.

Point six has to do with the body running a fever. What we're really made to believe is that a fever is a bad thing, it's not! Fevers are designed, number one, to tell us that the body is not working right, to take better care of ourselves. Number two, fevers are designed so that the body will cleanse. The fever helps the body to burn out toxins, and is necessary. Remember to drink plenty of fluids, and by that I mean water! Let the fever do its job.

Of course, if the fever gets too high we need to bring that fever down, but if we don't let the fever burn out those toxins, the toxins will keep backing up in the body, which will cause bigger health problems down the road.

*Sometimes a doctor is needed; sometimes medication is needed; just don't overdo it.

*The less toxins in the body, the less a person is sick. The less toxins, the milder are the health problems.

The more junk put into the body, the more intense the cold or cleansing. The purer the body, the gentler the cold or cleansing. The less toxins in the body the stronger the immune system. The less toxins in the body, the less the body is open to disease.

*Again, it is a very good possibility that the flu is an intense cleansing. The body is on overload.

Dis – Ease = Disease = Out Of Balance

What I am explaining is how to bring the body back to balance. Another word for balance is harmony.

Point seven is about sleep. To be able to sleep easily is a normal human function. It's not supposed to be difficult. It's not supposed to be hard. We shouldn't need sleeping pills or alcohol in order to go to sleep. It should be easy to do. Whether the lights in the house are on or off, we should be able to go to sleep. It's not about the mattress or the pillow, although a comfortable mattress and pillow is nice to have. It's about whether the body and mind is in balance, harmony.

Certainly, eating late at night is not a very good idea if you want to get a comfortable sleep. It's not a great idea to have caffeinated substances such as coffee and tea, or chocolate, as they rev the body up. How can a person go to sleep easily when they are taking stimulants during the day. It's a good idea to eat in moderation. To overeat makes it difficult to go to sleep, although most of us, today, overeat. To eat around five or six o'clock for dinner is a good time. Drink plenty of water, but not before you go to sleep, unless necessary.

What people do is they take uppers in the morning such as coffee, and maybe throughout the day, and then drink alcohol at night. Uppers and downers, taking the whole body, especially the nervous system on a roller coaster ride. Then we expect to be able to go to sleep easily. It just doesn't work that way.

Natural and refreshing sleep is a very important way for the body to do it's thing. I believe the less toxic a person is, the less sleep is needed to detoxify the body.

Other factors that have to do with natural and refreshing sleep are proper exercise and positive living, which will be discussed in book 2 and book 3.

A person has to play by the rules of the game of life, in order to be happy and healthy.

I've discussed how the body gets rid of waste, toxins, in a normal way. If we eat a proper diet; if we eat mostly food that is good for us, the body will get rid of waste through normal channels. Our immune system will be strong. Very rarely will we ever get sick. If we eat mostly a vegetarian diet, that means very little meat or dairy, or even a vegan diet, which is no meat or dairy at all, then the body will be healthy. When we're healthy we're playing by the rules of the game, because the body is functioning properly. The body is always trying to balance itself out. We've made it very easy for the body to do that.

By having a wonderful diet, very little cleansing is needed.

So, this is what happens; this is why we get sick. We've had plenty of warning signs such as headaches, stuffy nose, indigestion, dandruff, constipation, and we haven't listened. We've turned the headaches off with aspirin. We stopped the indigestion with antacids. We've used dandruff shampoo to stop the dandruff. We've taken enemas, or suppositories sometimes, or we just are constipated not going to the bathroom for days. The body is

15

just holding back more and more stuff. The body becomes overloaded. It becomes so backed up with waste, so loaded with toxins, that it's ready to explode. If it doesn't get rid of these toxins, this waste, this debris, the body will get sicker and sicker, and continue to deteriorate. It's as simple as that!

The body is getting all clogged up. We're taking all kinds of medication to stop the cleansing. Not only are we stopping the cleansing, we're putting more toxins into the body to stop it. What a disaster. My famous, Oh Brother!

You have to be smarter than the average bear!

Remember what I said, you're not sick, you are getting all clogged up.

Read on,

read on,

please, please, please,

read on!

I'm not so sure that I said this anywhere in the book so I'm saying it here. It's very possible that drinking more water will solve the problem of dry mouth and dry eyes. I know for myself that dry mouth disappeared when I increased my water intake. It's possible medication can cause dry mouth, or at least that's what they say. The better one takes care of themselves the less medication should be needed.

We're not playing by the rules of the game, the ones that work. We're playing by man-made rules, things that make profit for businesses. Finally, over time, the body is getting so clogged up, and breaking down more and more. More colds, more illnesses, more everything. The immune system is getting weaker and weaker.

The body's been breaking down for quite some time, begging for help. We're not listening! So over time, and that over time is happening at a younger and younger age, heart attacks, cancer, alzheimer's, etc., etc., etc. The body is suffocating in its own waste.

It's just common sense, what you put into the body has to come out. If it doesn't come out it has to be stored! The body is literally getting clogged up from years of neglect to the eyes, to the colon, to the arteries, to you name it. Everything is getting clogged up! I believe that hearing loss as we get older is due to the body getting clogged. I believe that macular degeneration is happening because the body has been getting clogged for a long time. Of course, high blood pressure, floaters in the eyes, all of these things may be just because the body is getting clogged. While the body doesn't look like it, it's slowly disintegrating.

This can be reversed, but we have to work on it, and not give up. You cannot give up! What I say is true, and the way to heal, works!

****

The body has been telling us to take better care of ourselves for years and we haven't listened, until hopefully now. Like I said earlier, if we work on it, our problems can be reversed! It takes a lot of years of determination, but I can tell you from my own experience that the body will reverse itself and get healthy. You may start to even notice the difference within a few weeks. The immune system will get stronger. Most of your problems will disappear or go into remission over time. That's what book 1, book 2, and book 3 are all about. How to play by the rules of the game. We're told that we have genetic weaknesses. Well, maybe we do; so what! Those so-called genetic weaknesses don't have to happen. There just weaknesses. Remember that for most of us God doesn't make, so-called, defective bodies, man does!

So, what do we do? How can you change your life, to feel better? Well, my question to you is; have you been kicked enough? Are you listening yet? Are you now willing to make a change? If you are, there's still time, even with so-called fatal diseases, to reverse your problems. Over the years, I've met many people that have reversed major health issues. From dandruff, to cancer, and everything in between. What I've seen, what I've heard, and what I believe, most health issues can be reversed. You have to believe, make a commitment to change your life, and do not give up. The key is, not to give up / Do Not Quit.

You have to change your lifestyle. I know it can be done, because I changed mine. I went from all types of meat, dairy products galore, and junk in general, to being almost a vegetarian. I take that back. I'm not almost a vegetarian; I'm closer to being a vegan. In fact, it's taken me so long to write this book, and get it out to you that I'm now a vegan. I have no animal products and almost no dairy. (I guess if somebody wants to be technical, because I have a tiny piece of cheese once in a while, I guess someone can find fault.)

Again, I know this can be done because I did it, and I know what can be done, because I did it. The first thing I did was to start to read the label of ingredients on packaged food, and to learn how to read it properly. I can tell you that food is labeled to confuse you in many cases. I have to believe though, that the ingredients section tells the truth; at least it's supposed to. I bought a nutrition book to show me the breakdown of food. What foods had iron in them. What foods had calcium. What foods had protein, and so forth and so on. At the time there were very few health food stores. I started to shop in them, more often than not. I bought the best quality food that I could afford, a lot of fresh fruits and vegetables, but because I didn't know very much, I have to admit, I sure made a lot of mistakes. I didn't give up! I didn't give up, and don't you give up either, because this works!!!. What I am telling you is, this absolutely works!

I went on a fast. I didn't know much about fasting and it lasted for about five days. I actually started to feel much better, but about four days into the fast I got diarrhea. Later, I found out that diarrhea not only will cause dehydration, but it's an extremely quick way for the body to release that stored garbage. It's a very fast way for the body to detoxify and can be dangerous. If you are going to fast for more than one or two days, it's my suggestion that you go to a doctor that knows how to help you through a fast. In fact, it's not a suggestion, I believe it's a necessity. I'll talk about fasting, later in this book.

It's not easy to eat healthy. There's so much junk food always around us, in pretty colors and pretty packaging. It took me a long time to totally change my diet. As I ate better and better food, the better I felt. The reason it took so long is I was a huge meat eater and dairy eater. My intestines must have really been clogged, because I guess I couldn't absorb enough nutrients from real food. Over time, I gradually cut back on meat and dairy. I was able to start absorbing the nutrition. Some people absorb the nutrition much faster. It didn't work that way for me, but I just wouldn't give up, because I knew it was the right direction to take. Almost immediately my dandruff disappeared. It came back a couple of times, slightly for a day or two, and then it disappeared. When I eat the wrong foods it might show up again. If it does, I know I've gone off my diet. As long as I eat a healthy diet, which means almost no meat or dairy, I have no dandruff.

My indigestion disappeared, the yellow around my eyes disappeared, my psoriasis disappeared. My extremities used to be cold, that stopped. My circulation increased, my sinus headaches were gone, and in general I felt much better. I have taken almost no medication for the past 30 years. I have run two low grade fevers in the beginning of changing my lifestyle. I consider both fevers to be very important, because I know without any doubt that my body was cleansing; burning out toxins. <u>Notice I say low grade fevers. Do not mess around with a high fever. You need to see a doctor.</u>

I finally, over a long time, cut out coffee. Sodas were easy to get rid of, but not coffee. I was addicted to the upper. In fact, I needed coffee every day.

Today, I wake up and I'm not tired. I sleep well. I don't need coffee to wake me up in the morning. I no longer have chocolate. My last big addiction is donuts which I am working very hard to break. Little by little that will be gone too. I don't miss any of the things I used to eat. There is so much good food to choose from, and my taste buds have changed, so real food tastes so much better. As my diet got purer I stop drinking alcohol completely. I just don't want it anymore! It seems the more balanced you become, the more the cravings stop. It's taken me so long to write this book, I look at a donut now and just don't want it. That's the darn truth. Just saying that makes me laugh. That craving has finally stopped. It was very important for me to kick coffee. I'll explain that a little later in this book. Don't let me forget.

I've got an interesting thought for you. When we exhale, what gas do we exhale? We have to get rid of that gas. Its carbon dioxide and the body can't use it. Plants love it, but it's not good for us. Okay, then think about this one. We drink sodas. Sodas have bubbles in them. What are those bubbles? You guessed it, carbon dioxide; gas the body can't wait to get rid of. We get hyper from the caffeine in some of the sodas; hyper from the sugar in some of the sodas. Then we get sluggish from the bubbles that are carbon dioxide. Now you tell me if we're using good sense! Boy oh boy! We must be nuts! The problem is until somebody told me this, I wouldn't have thought of it. I just thought you might be interested. It's so ridiculous. What a laugh.

So here we are. We've talked about how the body cleanses. If we allow the body to do what it's supposed to do, the body will detoxify. It just takes time for the body to cleanse itself. Gradually, over time, many of your problems will start to disappear. I can tell you that you can't give up. I can tell you that you can't get down on yourself, just keep going. I can tell you that you don't go straight forward. This is not the easiest road to take, but I will tell you, that over time, you'll be happy you did. Your brain will crave the old junky food, and once in a while you'll have to let yourself eat it. Don't get upset with yourself. Get on the right path as soon as you can. You will definitely start to feel better within a few weeks, maybe sooner. You may start to feel better in a few days. The more you do this, what I call proper eating, the more you will feel better! Over time you will not want to go back to the old you. The reason is, you'll like the new you much better. Some of your problems will get somewhat better. Some of your problems will go into remission, and some of your problems will disappear. Do not give up. Make a commitment to yourself to change your lifestyle, give yourself a great pat on the back, and put a smile on your face. I can tell you that, one day, the people that tell you you're crazy, hopefully they will ask you what you've done, and you can now teach them. I can tell you that from experience, because this works so well, you will want to help other people do what you've done. You will never gain weight again. You will feel so much better. You will look so much better, and you will like yourself so much more.

Let me tell you a story. I think we've all heard about the salmon. That's right the fish. Their stories amazing. They're born upstream. They swim towards the ocean and one day they get to the ocean. When I was younger, I was told in school that the people didn't know where the salmon were, once they got to the ocean. They stayed in the ocean for a certain amount of years, from what I remember. Then like clockwork they decide to go home. To do a cycle of birth that's been going on for a long, long time. So they swim back to that stream where they were born. They are determined to reach the point of their birth. They don't give up! They keep driving forward, under all kinds of conditions, they won't give up. They are determined to reach their goal.

In anything that we do in life, if we want to be successful, we can't give up. Sometimes, when we give up, success is just around the corner. Other fish probably tell the salmon that they're crazy. But, they know what they want, and they achieve their goal. They give it everything they've got. Put on blinders like a racehorse. Listen to your heart, and go for it. Not only will that salmon story help you with your health, it will help you with your life. I hope you like that story. It sure made an impression on me.

I understand, that at this point you probably are saying to yourself, I get the salmon story. It makes sense to me. But I still need help! I understand that. I am working on a website so I can help you. I will be doing some interactive conversations. I'm not a technology person, but I know you need help. I needed help too. The website is called YogaMattAcademy.com. At the end of the book there'll be more information, so that I can help you realize your dream of feeling great, looking great and thinking great.

Read on!

Okay! What Do I Do? What Do I Eat?

When I got started, as I said earlier, I knew nothing! The more I learned, the more I wanted to learn. How come I didn't know this? How come I didn't learn this in school? I guess some people tried to tell me, especially my father. I wasn't ready to listen. Hopefully you are now.

These are the fundamentals, basics:

One – Learn how to read the ingredients label on the back of the product you are buying. It is the only place you will get the truth of what the product truly is. Whatever they say on the rest of the product may, or may not be the truth. You'll notice that fresh fruits and vegetables need no ingredients label, because they are real food. Also, things such as raisins and pumpkin seeds, beans and grains, will just have on the ingredients label just what they are, and nothing else. What a breath of fresh air. Just food!

(Yellow raisins have a preservative in them. Watch out. Don't be fooled.)

Hippocrates said, let food be thy medicine, let medicine be thy food.

I can't understand it. The medical profession takes the Hippocratic Oath yet they know very little about nutrition. Listen to Hippocrates, he still knows what he's talking about.

Two – Get familiar with stores that sell quality food, such as grocery stores, health food stores, Asian stores, and Middle Eastern stores. Not only will the world open up to you on different types of food, but when you try these foods you will see that they are really great. Over time, your taste buds will taste real food. That real food will taste better and better. What you used to eat, in many cases, will taste poor to terrible. Over time, as you eat real food, and again that means fresh fruits, fresh vegetables, beans and grains, and nuts and seeds, your cravings will stop. Cravings such as coffee, or caffeinated tea, and junk food in general. The body won't want the garbage. In fact the body will know that the garbage food makes it sick. Smoking may actually stop as well, as the brain says, why are you doing this?

Three – Get a good nutrition book. A book that has the breakdown of nutritional values of food. You will find that there is plenty of protein, plenty of vitamins, plenty of calcium, plenty of iron, and plenty of everything else that you need. (Seeds, nuts, beans and grains, have plenty of protein. Fruits and vegetables, and the above are loaded with iron and calcium. Check out raisins and pumpkin seeds. You will be amazed at how much high quality nutrition is in wonderful, real food.)

Four – As I've said before, as your body starts to cleanse, the nutrition will be absorbed easier, which will allow you to have less animal products. (I would immediately start to cut way down your meat intake. That includes red meat, chicken, fish, eggs, etc. As stated earlier eat small portions of animal products, no more than about three times per week.) If you are going to eat animal products your best bet is to purchase the highest quality animal products you can find, such as organic meat. I say that because there are so many contaminants in meat today. Hormones and antibiotics, plus nobody even knows what's in the meat. Why anybody would allow female hormones to go into meat, or male hormones to go into meat; I just can't figure it out! It makes no sense. It's got to be dangerous. Get the purists meat you can get. Eat very little of it.

Five – Gradually cut out all dairy products, and I mean all. People are having way too much dairy and the fat is absolutely clogging up the body. You can't expect to cut dairy products out overnight, that I understand, but reduce them as quickly as you can. Dairy includes milk, cheese of any kind, yogurt of any kind, and ice cream of any kind. Low-fat milk is not a solution, because low-fat milk has more casein in it. Casein is thought to be the reason dairy causes osteoporosis. No matter which way you look at it, dairy is a problem. I believe dairy is the biggest reason that we have so many health issues today. (Dairy should be had sparingly, if eaten at all.)

Some of this next part is repetitious, but I think it's important to say again. It's a commandment that says: thou shall not kill. That commandment doesn't mean just people. It means anything that doesn't want to give up its life. We should respect all life. That means animals. That means everything. The earth is essentially alive. It just doesn't mean human beings. Plants give off oxygen. Trees being the biggest giver of oxygen. No oxygen, no us. Do we respect life? I can tell you that an animal doesn't want to give up its life. I can also tell you that eating animals, over time, will eventually destroy you. I think I said before, the strongest animal on the planet is the elephant. The elephant is a vegetarian. It's also the biggest animal. So size and strength have nothing to do with eating meat. When we kill and eat an animal their fear of dying and their anger also becomes part of us. It's probably one of the reasons were having so many problems in this country. The animals' adrenaline becomes ours. People are becoming immune to antibiotics, possibly because we're feeding so many antibiotics to the animals, to prevent them from getting sick.

Did you ever see a person with a big stomach? Why do you think that stomachs so big? Unless that person is pregnant, that person is probably loaded with meat and its fat. That meat and fat could be 20 years old, maybe more. It sits in the body and clogs it up. The intestines are distended. As you eat more garbage, especially meat, the stomach gets bigger and bigger until you can't even see your toes. Pretty gross isn't it? Next time when you drive down the street and you see an animal that's been killed, think about the animal that you eat. There is not much difference. That animal that you destroy today, I will tell you, will eventually destroy you. Makes you really think, doesn't it? What's coming out of you when you have a cold is animal, the preservatives, food dyes, and other junk. Garbage that the body can't use. Oh brother! Sometimes people just don't get sick. *They don't cleanse. You have to cleanse, so-called getting sick, so-called getting a*

cold. *Those are the people that say, I've been healthy my whole life, how did I get this major illness? Again, thank the person that gave you a cleansing, that triggered your body to release toxins.*

So now the question is, what about plants? We eat plants. Why are they okay to eat? We don't eat an apple tree, we eat the apple. We don't eat a peach tree, we eat a peach. The tree drops its food for us to eat. There are many plants that will die sooner if we don't take its food. Plants want you to take their food. The world is amazing. Take a cucumber, you'll get more cucumbers. Plants are very generous to give us their food.

Think about what's happening to all of us, especially the young people. We don't have defective bodies, in most cases. We are putting terrible fuel into our body. To be healthy the fuel needs to change.

You know, when I was a kid, we were taught the two most important food groups were meat and dairy. We were conned! We were had!

> *The human being truly only needs milk when it's in its infancy, and mother's milk is still far and above the best.*

This is why! Mother's milk is for human consumption. Cow's milk is for a baby cows consumption. Goat's milk is for goats consumption. I think that makes perfect common sense. All of the above have milk that is formulated for their own kind. Human milk has just the right amount of everything to not only nourish the baby, but in the early years, protect the baby. That's why it's so important for the mother and the father to eat a good diet, so not only is the baby healthy, but the mother's milk is also as healthy as possible.

Again, what we are feeding the animal, in most cases, is not only making the animal extremely sick, but it is also doing the same thing to us. We are killing the animal, and the animal is slowly destroying us.

Six – When you read the ingredients label on packaged food, anything you do not understand, usually means don't buy the product. Your best bet is to buy mostly from the fresh fruits and vegetables section, anyhow.

Seven – Stay away from foods that have dye additives. The food may look pretty, but it's not real food. The food manufacturer makes it colorful, so that you will buy their product. Real foods, that are used as dye, are okay. You must understand the words. For instance, beets give a dark purple color.

Eight – Stay away from all sodas, plus other junk. Sodas are loaded with sugar, or synthetic sweeteners, and bubbles of carbon dioxide. Remember my earlier story about carbon dioxide. It is a toxic gas which the body must get rid of. Start to cut down your addiction to chocolate candy, coffee and caffeinated teas. Be very careful when food companies tell you that these products are good for you. They are addictive and harmful. Over time believe it or not you will get rid of these products almost entirely. Caffeinated products push water out of the body. They are diuretics and may cause people to become dehydrated. (Caffeinated products are an upper, definitely speeds up the body, and helps to screw up the nervous system. No wonder people can't sleep.)

Nine – Stop drinking, or cut way, way back, all alcoholic beverages. Beer pushes water out of the body. It has to create dehydration because you pee more than you take in. Just my own common sense says it has to be tough on the kidneys. Be careful of wine. It's a downer, as probably most alcoholic beverages are. People that have caffeine that's in coffee, chocolate, sodas, all day and then wine at night; oh brother! That stuff has got to screw you up really bad. In fact, doing that will cause major health issues. Again people are taking uppers and downers. Eventually, moving the nervous system out of control. To me, it's like taking legalized drugs. Then you want to have a good night sleep? As my friend from New York says, Forget About It.

I will tell you from my own experience that as you eat better food. As your body gets back into balance again. You will want less alcohol. You will eventually stop drinking altogether!

Ten – Stay away from preservatives the best you can. Not only are those preservatives preserving the food, they are also preserving you. Be careful of oils that don't make sense, such as cottonseed oil. I'm not so sure that I can eat cotton. Laugh out loud. Oh brother!

Eleven – Drink plenty of healthy, wonderful, beautiful, clean water! Distilled water, reverse osmosis water, filtered water, and maybe springwater. The purer the water, the more the water will leach toxins out of the body. At home I drink reverse osmosis water. I buy distilled water or reverse osmosis water when on a trip. When I'm in a restaurant, I hope that the water will be okay. (You can generally tell if the water is not filtered. It tastes terrible.)

It's very possible that drinking more water will solve the problem of dry mouth and dry eyes. I know for myself that dry mouth disappeared when I increased my water intake. It's possible medication can cause dry mouth, or at least that's what they say. The better one takes care of themselves the less medication should be needed.

I wanted to explain something about me. I'm not a writer, I'm not an author, I'm a thinker. My sister says; where did I come from? We're so much alike, my sister and me, yet were so different. What I talk about in this book just pores out of me. I've helped so many people because I can't stand to watch what's going on with the health and happiness of people. Sometimes the book gets repetitive, I know that. I'm trying to put the book into an order that makes sense to you. This stuff just pores out of me. So, I hope you will understand when sometimes things seem out of order, or I've said it before. I've never met any of you, but I feel for all of you. I want your life to be better, happier and healthier. I genuinely care. Don't ask me why it's important to me, it just is! What no one understands is this is what makes me tick. I know I can help people. I'm not a doctor but I have helped so many people that doctors can't help. I have helped people where doctors wanted to perform surgery. I have just plain helped people! So, let's go on with the book and I hope you'll understand that this all comes from my heart.

The High-Cost Of Medical Insurance

take charge of your life, stay healthy

The cost of medical insurance has gone out of control. I think about that a lot. When The Affordable Care Act was passed, better known as Obama

Care, I knew there had a be problems. I said it would break the bank. The reason I believed that nobody could afford it was the fact that we never addressed the problem. It's like we want people to be sick. If people are sick there is an awful lot of people that make an awful lot of money. Let me list some of them; pharmaceutical companies, drug stores, doctors, nurses, hospitals, the crap food industry. There's an awful lot of money to be made. The expression is, follow the money. If we really do want people to be healthy, the first thing we need to do is to concentrate on cleaning up the food industry. I believe there is a good reason for the medical profession and food industry to exist, but not to the extent that we are using them. If people took charge of their life, and stopped buying junk food all the above industries would go into decline, or have to change in a far better way. The people that are getting rich, on the people getting sick, would make far less money, or be out of a job.

Now we have a new government administration, and we will have a new medical insurance plan. How can it work? We still haven't addressed the main reason why people are sick! It's mostly the food. How loud can I say it! The costs will still keep going out of control.

You have to take charge of your life. If you don't, the above will take charge of it for you. (Remember, you are no good to the medical profession if you are healthy.

It almost appears as if the medical profession wants to keep you sick, and make you sicker. Be smarter than the average bear, that means take charge of your life. Eat healthier food, a better exercise program, and a better way to keep the mind happy. (I will discuss a better exercise program, and a better way to keep the mind healthy and happy, in the two books to follow.)

Obesity

I touched on obesity briefly. Obesity needs to be discussed as an extremely important issue. We are trying to make obesity glamorous, but it's not. The medical profession calls obesity a disease, but it's not. I do not believe that obesity, for most of us, is a genetic weakness. Obesity is a problem that can be solved.

I talk in this book about a proper diet. Proper diet means eating good, quality food. I'm not talking about going on a diet just to lose weight. I'm talking about a lifestyle change. The reason that people go on a so-called diet and lose weight is because they're essentially eating a lot less calories and possibly starving the body. Also, they're probably doing more exercise. When they break the diet they go back up in weight, sometimes higher than they were before. I watch people make fortunes off of diet books. I watch people that are sicker than hell make fortunes off of diet and exercise books. If you go to a doctor to lose weight, why would you go to a doctor that weighs 200 pounds and is only five feet tall? That's what people do! Oh brother! People let somebody else cook for them and send dehydrated food in the mail. First of all we learned nothing, and secondly, is that food they cook for us, really any good for us. If you want to lose weight learn how to truly lose weight. Learn how to do it yourself. Learn how to take better care of yourself. One of the things that I've noticed is that people are getting heavier, and truthfully, some don't even know why. I know that seems hard to believe, but I believe it's true. Keeping your weight down means making a lifestyle change. If you do it long enough, it becomes automatic. And because you like yourself so much better, and because you are now on a new path, you will keep your weight off; never to be heavy again. You have to make a commitment to yourself, and you have to keep that commitment.

People that are overweight are prone to many health issues. If you read this book over and over again, you will start to change your life. You will eventually eat a proper diet. You will eventually do a great exercise. You will eventually have a happy life. I can assure you that book 2 and book 3 will follow. This is my commitment to you, and to me. Again, to help you makes me happy. I will not let you down.

Many people spent a lot of time teaching me, putting up with my stuff, and made a huge, positive difference in my life. At the end of this book will be a coupon. This coupon will entitle you to internet classes, helping you to reinforce how to eat properly, how to exercise properly, and how to be just plain happier. First month just 5.00. The website will be:

YogaMattAcademy.com

This is my dream, to help you help yourself, so that you can look better, feel better, think better, and be better. I want to help you learn how to play by the rules of the game of life.

This is what my father used to say, don't overeat, and eat everything in moderation. For most of his life he did exactly that. I read in a book; the quickest way to dig your grave is through your teeth. My father lived to be three months shy of 100 years old. I think I said in this book earlier he was my first teacher. My father was a big believer in anticancer foods. He was right, he would talk about broccoli. But there are more; collards, kale, parsley, dark leafy green vegetables. He would say moderation with moderation. My dad would have a soda once in a while. My dad would have ice cream once in a while; only a single scoop. He would eat a very small amount of meat. My dad was not a big eater.

My father didn't know everything; neither do I, but he made terrific suggestions. He would say dilute your juice. Too much sugar in orange juice. He would add probably 25 percent juice to 75 percent water. Not a bad idea. My father got macula degeneration at 88 years old. Today with what I now know, I think I could've helped him. I think it was those damn french fries he would eat in restaurants. Too much altered fat and maybe not enough water. I'll never know for sure, but I'd sure like a chance to help other people with the same problem, to see if I was right.

My father also created his own exercise program, some of which I intend to teach. My father would exercise every day. His exercise was gentle. Not this intense exercise that we see today. This intense exercise is breaking the body down over time. More of that in book 2.

****

Be careful of those high acid foods, such as coffee, tomato sauce or tomato juice, and orange juice, etc. My suggestion is to eliminate coffee altogether. Tomato juice and orange juice is pure acid, on top of that orange juice is loaded with sugar. Do you know how many oranges or tomatoes it takes to make a tall glass of juice? You would never eat that many of the whole fruit, at one sitting. Plus, the enzymes are missing, which balance out the fruit. When you heat the food the enzymes are destroyed. That's probably one of the reasons why the oriental people use a wok. Most people have a tendency to melt the food.

Why do I suggest staying off caffeine products? Number one, caffeine products are addictive. Number two, they burn out the adrenal glands. You know what adrenaline is? Adrenaline gives you an extra surge if you need to run, or maybe lift something heavy that you normally couldn't do. I remember my mother many years ago, lifting my niece who had been stung by a bee. My mother was small. My niece was probably about 60 or 70 pounds at the time. My mother carried my niece effortlessly, probably 300 yards from the swimming pool to the house. My mother didn't have that kind of strength; she did then, adrenaline. I have heard about a person that could lift a car slightly to free another person from under the car, adrenaline. Adrenaline is important and when we have caffeine products we slowly deteriorate the adrenal glands, so we have less and less energy. So we need to stimulate the body more and more and more. Coffee, more chocolate, more sodas, maybe more tea. Be careful of caffeine. In the stores today they sell small bottles loaded and I mean loaded with caffeine, be careful! Our nervous system is being decimated, and we are slowly destroying ourselves. Eventually, we can't even wake up without a stimulant, such as coffee. We need the energy boost all throughout the day. Kicking caffeine is not easy. I can tell you though, that you will kick the drug, caffeine, if you are determined to do it. It takes time, but it is worth it. No wonder so many people are drinking wine. We're either f lying, or inebriated. Uppers and downers, taking the body on a roller coaster ride. (By the way regular tea ain't so great either. Kick the habit, you'll be a lot happier you did. Drink herbal tea, that's the way to go.)

As you slowly cut down your coffee, I will tell you that you will go through some withdrawals. You'll probably get headaches for a couple of days, and I can't tell you what else, but you just have to accept that the body is craving the coffee. In a couple of days you won't get those headaches, and whatever else that was happening should stop too. You will still feel that you need your coffee because you're going to be tired without it. Gradually over time your energy will come back as your body starts to get stronger, and as it does you won't want coffee or chocolate or sodas. Find another way to wake up. Do a little exercise; take a cool shower or go for a brisk walk. If you are getting palpitations, those will eventually stop. If your heart is skipping from all the caffeine, drink more water. I know that there is a lot to remember. This is not going to happen overnight, but if you don't give up, you will get there, and you will feel better; Much Better!

I said before, I know I'm repeating myself, one of the leading causes of osteoporosis is dairy products. The next is animal products and the next is caffeine products. We are pushing way too many dairy products on the women. Just wait till you see the osteoporosis in women at an early age. You ain't seen nothin yet.

Try to have a pizza without cheese. Lots of fresh vegetables, maybe a little pineapple with a little bit of tomato sauce; no cheese. It will taste the same! Most people don't even notice the difference. I can tell you the second time you eat it, it will taste great. Give it a try!

Cut back on the meat, but if you get a hamburger, get it without cheese. Too much fat, too much protein, too much junk.

For breakfast get one egg, potatoes or grits, and toast. Be careful of the oil, the butter or margarine. No cheese. Don't let people put a bunch of junk in front of you. Learn how to take charge of your life.

Young men and women are getting sick from all the crap we're putting into our body. Diseases that shouldn't be. Overweight that shouldn't be. Eating way too much junk. Young people, older people, everybody storing junk. It's not leaving the body. Children are storing junk, waste, toxins, at an alarming rate. If the mother's diet is bad, if the father's diet is bad, oh brother. As a society, you ain't seen nothin yet unless we change our lifestyle.

I was just watching a movie on television. In that movie the phrase was used, "miracles are everywhere." You are a miracle. You are entitled to be healthy. You are entitled to be happy.

Water

drink plenty of good clean water

Water, water everywhere, and people
are living as if they're in a desert.

Let's really talk about water. Drinking enough water is so, so important. The body is about 65 to 70 percent water. I keep saying that throughout the book. Drink plenty of good clean water. It's so important to understand, to know why. Every cell has water in it, and we all know that the blood is mostly liquid. These are my thoughts, these are my opinions, and these are my facts.

If the body dehydrates too much, we will die.

Read on

We can live longer without food, than we can without water. Water is essential to good health.

The bloodstream is like a river. That river carries nutrients to all parts of the body, and also removes toxins, waste, from all parts of the body. That waste comes out from the eyes, from the nose, from the pores, in the urine and in the stool. By drinking enough water the river flushes debris the way it should. Think of a river after a rainstorm. If it has not rained for many days that river will run slowly. Once it rains the river runs much faster. If it doesn't rain for a long time the river may eventually dry out.

I don't expect anybody to read this book in one day. But please finish the book. Reread the book. Forget about some of the duplication of information. I'm trying to get you to change your life. I know you will be healthier and I know you will be happier.

Again, think of the Grand Canyon. The Grand Canyon has the great Colorado River running right through it. Many believe that the Grand Canyon was created by that great Colorado River. It took a long time to carry that debris with it and that great, beautiful, wonderful, amazing Grand Canyon, without that wonderful healthy river, would have never existed. The same thing applies to us. Our river, our bloodstream carries with it nutrients and waste. Drinking plenty of good clean water allows our river, our bloodstream, to do its job properly. Please listen. What I'm saying in this book will put a smile on your face!

Years ago I went to a class talking about water. This is what I heard that to me was really important. The purer the water, the faster the waste can be carried out of the body. That's why I say drink plenty of good clean water. I've mentioned I use reverse osmosis water at home. When I'm out I do the best I can. I'm not a fanatic. When I go on a trip I buy distilled water or reverse osmosis water in gallon containers. I don't like buying water in plastic. I can't be a fanatic. You have to do the best you can. (Buying water for the home in plastic makes no sense.) The purer the water the more it gets rid of waste. Water sitting in plastic containers will eventually leach the plastic into the water. The best container for water is glass, do the best you can. I want people to think about what they're doing, that's the reason I wrote this book. I want to make a positive difference in your life. Contact YogaMattAcademy.com. Let me know how you're doing! You have to be improving if you're doing what this book is talking about. You have to get better! I will be doing streaming. I will be doing conference calling if I can figure out how to do it to try to keep you on the right track and try to answer your questions. I know this can be done because I did it. You have the power to be a happy camper, to put a smile on your face and a song in your heart. Oh well, enough of that!

Let's go on. You'll find this information very interesting.

A friend of mine sent the following to me many, many years ago. As I'm writing this book it popped up again. It's one of the pieces that made me stop and think. I hope it does the same for you.

75 percent of Americans are chronically dehydrated.

In 37 percent of Americans, the thirst mechanism is so weak that it is often mistaken for hunger.

One glass of water will shut down midnight hunger pangs for almost 100 percent of the dieters studied, in a university study.

Lack of water, the number one trigger of daytime fatigue.

Preliminary research indicates that 8 to 10 glasses of water a day will significantly ease back and joint pain for up to 80 percent of sufferers.

A mere two percent drop in body water can trigger fuzzy short-term memory; trouble with basic math and difficulty focusing on the computer screen or on a printed page.

Drinking five glasses of water daily decreases the risk of colon cancer by 45 percent, plus it can decrease the risk of breast cancer by 79 percent, and one is 50 percent less likely to develop bladder cancer.

<u>*Make Sure That You Drink Enough, Good
Clean, Healthy Water, Every Day!*</u>

I'm just thinking here; a little bit of knowledge. Two of the more balanced foods that I know of, are apples and brown rice. Sometimes, I think about roughage from fruits and vegetables, especially grains, especially brown rice. I feel it's possible the roughage somehow allows the blood to have a little bit of a grit. A very mild scrubbing agent, that keeps the arteries clean. I've never read that anywhere, but I believe that, that's very possible. I know that I've read somewhere that brown rice depletes the body of fat. I know that's possible. If you can, I suggest that you eat brown rice 2 to 3 times a week. It has B vitamins, it's a balanced food. I think brown rice is great. Apples are an outstanding fruit. They can be mixed with vegetables because they're very balanced, and apples are loaded with enzymes. Just remember it's all about eating real food. (I suggest that you mix brown rice with a small amount of millet. Like five percent millet to brown rice. The small amount of millet balances out the brown rice. It prevents brown rice from being too acidic.) The easiest way to cook brown rice and most grains is in a pressure cooker. You've probably heard of millet, birds eat it. I happen to love millet, and I'm not a bird. You may love it too.

I have heard it said, that the blood of a plant is the chlorophyll. Green vegetables, dark leafy green vegetables are very healthy for you. There are so many people that don't eat vegetables. I would say that they get sick more often. The reason being the body will become very toxic from what they are eating. (When people eat food with empty nutrition, people eat more food. That may be one of the reasons why people are so heavy. Makes sense to me.)

****

READ ON

As I said earlier, get a good nutrition book. This is extremely important. One that breaks down nutrition by calories, by protein and by nutrients, etc. A book that has a good nutritional chart. Put the book somewhere so you can read it every day. Look at the nutritional breakdown of fresh fruits and fresh vegetables. Look at all of it, including seaweed. Get an idea of the value of food.

In the above paragraph I mentioned the word seaweed. Seaweed has great nutrition in it. It has a lot of iodine, it has protein, it has B vitamins, etc. If you don't have iodized salt in the house, and you don't eat seafood, you're not getting iodine unless you have seaweed. The main reason for iodine is to prevent a goiter, the swelling in the neck. I eat seaweed because of the iodine, and because now I like it. When I first tried seaweed I thought I was going to die from it. It tasted awful. In fact, I threw it in the garbage, then I said, let me try again. This time it wasn't so terrible. It wasn't the seaweed, it was my taste buds, and the fact that I've never tasted seaweed before. As my taste buds got healthier, the food tasted better. You can actually, eventually, taste food. I really like seaweed such as dulse, which is a good source of iodine. I like nori, which is used in Japanese vegetable rolls, so you may already be eating seaweed. What really happened is I now love real food!

Food is amazing; beautiful colors and textures. Just think of it, out of one pumpkin come 200 to 300 seeds. Enough seeds to grow hundreds and hundreds of pumpkins. Out of one tomato come many seeds. Those many seeds can grow hundreds of tomatoes. Real food is amazing.

**(Just a thought, most fish is farmed fish.
Be careful what you eat today.)**

Somewhere in this book I mentioned learning how to read the ingredients label on packaged food. By this, I mean canned food, boxed food, food in paper or cellophane. The only label, as I've said before, that means anything, is the ingredients label. The first ingredient is the most important in the product. The second is the second most important ingredient. The third ingredient is the third most important, and so on. If there are things you cannot understand, in an ingredients label, it's a warning sign. Do not buy the product! It's generally a preservative. It's not good for you whatever it is. Don't buy the food. Preservatives, preserve you too. Stay away from MSG and any name that they use that is MSG, which are quite a few. Stay away from all those altered foods and fats. Stay away from the poison that companies are trying to sell you. Stay away from the colored food that makes the food look pretty, unless it is natural. Read the ingredients label. Some of the packaged food that companies tell you is food, is nothing but junk. It has very little food value at all. To me, it's like eating a plastic plate. Be careful, for some reason the food industry seems to want to destroy us. Stay away from baked goods that are sitting out too long. Most of them have preservatives like crazy in them. Not only do I believe preservatives preserve you; I also believe they cannot come out of the body easily and so they add to your weight and certainly to a person getting sick. They are poison, toxic. They will destroy you over time. Try to buy almost everything you can from the fresh fruits and vegetables section, as I've said before. Try to buy organic. If organic is not affordable, buy the best food you can. Stay away from the toxic food. Read the ingredients label. Some food that is packaged is okay; read the ingredients. The word on the rest of the package can say anything. It is the ingredients label, according to law, that must be accurate. That is the best you can do. (Sometimes, I wonder if the ingredients label is accurate, just do the best you can.)

I was just looking at the back of a can of organic pumpkin. We use it to make pumpkin pie sometimes. In the back of the can are the nutritional facts. Almost all products list the facts the same way. Here's what the label says: first, serving size. Be careful there, because companies are trying to fool you. They give different serving sizes: in tablespoons, cups, one half cup, one quarter cup, and a full cup, etc. Make sure you know the serving size first. Then comes servings per container. Next calories, this is where it's important to know the serving size. One half cup has 100 calories, versus one quarter teaspoon has 100 calories. The nutritional facts: saturated fat, trans fat, cholesterol and sodium. It's really important to know how many calories per serving size. It's also important to know the percentage of carbohydrates and fiber, sugar, protein and vitamins. It is very important to know both the nutritional facts when you buy the products, and the ingredients. Many of the foods that you are buying now will have a lot of calories, but they are weak, or empty of nutrition. If food is weak, in nutrition, it's possible, like I said earlier, we need more food, because we are trying to get enough nutrition. Again, this is the reason why people may be gaining weight. It took me a long time to understand all this information. You will get it over time. Sometimes, I still get fooled. Do not give up!

Salad dressing has little to no nutritional value, but it's extremely high in empty calories. It's amazing how many processed foods are empty of nutrition. Please, please, please, read the ingredients label. That label will change your life.

If you are buying a can of food, try to buy a can that is not dented. The reason that you buy a can that is not dented, is because the can is made of aluminum and has a plastic lining. It's possible that the aluminum will seep into the food. The lining of the plastic may be broken. Also, do not scrape the can. Use a soft something to get the last of the food out. I'm not so crazy about food being in plastic, either! If possible buy food that is in a glass container.

What Is Cancer

I want to digress a little. I was just listening to a television commercial. We've been working on the cure for cancer for a long, long time. We've been working on major diseases for a long, long time. What is cancer? Early in this book, I mentioned I knew quite a few people that have cured themselves of cancer. I've also listened to doctors explain things that made sense to me about this terrible disease. I've listened at least to one doctor that cured herself of cancer.

Well, what is cancer? When a person gets sick they just don't let the body cleanse. We stop the cleansing. We get that so called cold. We stop the nose from running. We bring that fever down. We take an aspirin to stop the headache but we never address the issue. We never allow the body to cleanse. We stop everything. We stop the armpits from sweating. We go to the gym to work out, and we can hardly sweat because the gym is cold.

We have terrible diets and we put toxic food into our body. We never let the poison come out. We are constipated beyond belief because people don't eat a lot of fruits and vegetables. There's very little water in the food they eat, and certainly people do not drink enough water. What do we expect? Eventually the body has got to give out. We are going completely out of balance. A major disease, such as cancer has to happen. You can't put garbage into the gas tank and expect the car to run; it won't do that. In fact the car doesn't just stop running; it dies. Other major diseases such as Alzheimer's, and heart disease are probably happening for the same reason. The body is clogging up. The body is fighting for survival.

People get fibromyalgia, a disease that nobody can find. The body is toxic, it can't move. You don't have to be a rocket scientist to figure this out. You don't have to be a doctor to figure this out. You've got to use common sense. Water in the gas tank causes the car to stop running. If you don't change the oil in the car, that car will eventually turn to junk. What are people thinking? I'm not against medication. I go to a doctor when I need one. I like to eat some lousy food once in a while. Notice, I said once in a while. If I eat junk every day, I will get sicker and sicker. My body's cells will literally become more and more toxic. My body will have to cleanse, or as we say in this country, catch a cold. If I don't let my body cleanse the cells will eventually suffocate, because they will be so loaded with toxins. My body's cells will start to give out and if they do that's when a major disease will occur. My body is literally fighting to survive. The cells are backing up, they are dying, they can't breathe, they can't function. What are people thinking? Let the body cleanse. Bring real food, real nutrition into the body, and drink plenty of good clean water.

What they sell us in the stores is lots of junk. Pretty colored packaging, with lots of fake information on them to confuse us. Read the ingredients label. Do not get fooled! People have tons of coffee, alcohol, chocolate, junk, junk, junk. Like I said before, be very careful of dairy. I became a vegan, no dairy at all, but if you have dairy do it in small amounts. And if you're trying to heal cut the dairy out! The body is backing up and backing up and backing up. Backing up with toxins, begging you to stop eating the garbage. We get sick, we suppress the cold, the cleansing. The body can't get rid of the waste. We don't listen to our body. We don't take charge of our life. We give our power to other people. We give our power totally to the medical profession. Doctors know very little about nutrition. They give shots and pills. They make their big-money from surgery. I'm not against doctors, but I will tell you if you take care of yourself and you feed your body quality fuel, you'll see those doctors rarely. Remember about medication, it has terrible side effects and in some cases one of the side effects, and I've heard this quite a few times is death. Side effects of Alzheimer's medication sometimes is memory loss. Oh brother! Some of the medication is addictive so not only do we have a health problem, but now we become a drug addict. Doesn't it make sense to change your lifestyle? Don't turn your power over to somebody else. Please listen to your body, you can get healthy again. Let your body discharge, let your body detoxify, let your body cleanse; please!

Cancer is the body telling you, if you do not take care of your life right now; no more warnings, no more red lights. If you do not take care of your body right now, to let it cleanse, then the body is kaput, finished. Man, I haven't used the word kaput in a long, long time. I must really be on a roll.

When your body is healthy, we detoxify normally, because the body has so little waste. The cells do not have to go through an extreme discharge, and so we don't get sick. We detoxify gently. The immune system is strong, the body is healthy, that's just the way it is.

Please!!! Let your body throw off the toxins. Please!!! Let your body get rid of the waste.

Get out of survival and into happiness, please, please, please! Get into balance, get into harmony.

Book 2 and book 3 will have to do with get into laughter and get into a proper exercise program. Reduce stress. Learn how! (I'm not talking about antidepressants to reduce stress. Man, that word antidepressants is really a long word.)

Calories are energy. What kind of energy do you want to put into your body; your temple.

*Women check your makeup, it seals the pores. The face has to breathe. At least take the makeup off when you don't need it. I may have said this earlier in the book, buy high-quality, healthy makeup, please!

I used to go to a yoga retreat. I would notice that when the women came in, they were dressed to kill. Once they checked in, they would go to their room, change into some casual clothes and most would take their makeup off. They looked very different. In fact, I didn't recognize them, in some cases. After a few days that's who they were. For the most part those are the people that I knew, the casual people. Then when they got ready to leave they put their makeup on. I'm laughing as I'm writing this, because it's so ridiculous. Now I didn't recognize them again. They looked so different. Truthfully, I thought they looked very good without their makeup. Sometimes, I remember to shaking my head and saying, the world's nuts.

Years ago I had a hairpiece. What a pain in the neck. I don't know if I looked better, I certainly looked different. Once people got to know me with my hairpiece on, now I couldn't take it off. But I got sick and tired of it. So finally, after a while, I took it off. So now I didn't have my hairpiece. I thought people were going to notice and they were going to say boy, you sure look different. You know what, I don't think anybody noticed one way or the other. Oh yeah, one customer said to me, you look different, did you lose weight? So, people, take care of that body of yours. Women, wear as little makeup as you can.

Don't give up!
Read on...

Sugar
use common sense

The question is, is sugar bad for you? The answer is, no! It's not the sugar that's bad for you it's the way we have the sugar, that makes it bad for you. Take an orange, any orange. I said earlier, somewhere in this book that an orange is healthy. Oranges have nutrition in them, water in them, enzymes in them, that's good! But, having eight oranges at one sitting is not a great idea. Too much sugar, too much acid, and why in the world would someone have eight oranges at one sitting. That's what we do when we have a glass of orange juice. Would you ever eat eight oranges at one time? Squeeze a fresh squeezed glass of orange juice. A small glass is at least three oranges. Most people don't have a small glass of orange juice. If you are buying orange juice in a carton it's probably pasteurized, heated. Lots of acid, lots of sugar, no enzymes. The same thing goes for any juice, tomato juice, grapefruit juice, or any other kind of juice. Eat the fruit. Get the roughage, get the nutrition, get the enzymes, and enjoy the fruit. Sometimes not only do they process the juice, but then they add other stuff to it, vitamins for instance, maybe more sugar; what a joke! Eat the individual, real fruit.

Have you ever seen anyone get sweet tea. They must use tablespoons of sugar in that sweet tea. People do the same thing with coffee. Tons of sugar, concentrated, white sugar. The same thing happens with sodas. Tons and tons of sugar. I'll tell you one thing; manufacturers of that sugar really love you, and so does the dentist. Not only are we f lying from the caffeine, the upper, were also supporting our local dentist.

So, let's talk about white sugar. White sugar is processed. Well, how bad could that be? Do you know what a sugarcane looks like? It's tall and round. Believe it or not, you don't get much sugar out of one sugarcane. They have to squeeze it to get the sugar, and boil it to get rid of the water. So, when you have sugar, how many sugar canes are you eating to get that amount of sugar? I love real Maple Syrup. I mean real Maple Syrup. Maple Syrup comes from the sap of a tree. I remember as a little boy seeing how they make it. They boil the syrup, get rid of the water, and what's left is the Maple Syrup. Be careful these are concentrated sugars. Too much of this is dangerous to your health. Eat fresh fruit.

Remember to read the ingredients label.

**If you are going to buy Maple Syrup, buy the real thing.
Don't buy junk food, it will eventually destroy you.**

****

**Keep reading, don't just put this book on the shelf.
This book will change your life. You will be happier!
You will feel better! You will think better!**

Show this book to your friends. Make a difference in their life too!

Oil Is Fat In Liquid Form**

Let's talk about fat, or in liquid form oil. (When I say the word oil I mean fat. When I say the word fat I mean oil, because they are one and the same.)

Fat is calories; lots of calories. Fat is very high in calories! The less fat you eat the more weight you will lose, especially if you are eating fruits and vegetables, beans and grains. Remember, oil is fat!

There are three kinds of fat. One kind of fat is saturated fat. All oils have some saturated fat, but animal products generally have the most. Coconut Oil and Palm Oil are also high in saturated fat. Saturated fat does not come out of the body easily. It does not melt at room temperature. It stays in the body and clogs the body. It is easy to see a meat eater. Over time, that person will have a big stomach because they're holding on to the meat in their intestines, excuse me, not the meat, the animal's fat. Through eating a proper diet, that fat will eventually be pushed out of the body; it will be released. Possibly some of the mucous coming out of your body, out of your nose when you get a so called cold, is saturated fat. All kinds of dairy will do the same thing. The dairy, being high in saturated fat, will also clog up the body. Of course, if you eat meat, once in a while, you will cleanse through normal channels.

The second kind of fat, or oil, is hydrogenated fat. Hydrogenated fat is altered oil. Margarine is a hydrogenated oil. It's a corn oil, for instance, that has been altered, so it stays hard at room temperature. Manufacturers do that so you can spread it like butter. Hydrogenated oils also are not easy to leave the body, they also clog the body.

I have heard for many years, that oil, if re-cooked is not good for you. You know what? I believe that means all the chips, french fries that you buy anywhere, are probably not good for you. Be careful of what you eat! You can check reused oil and its problems on the internet. I used to go to a Japanese restaurant; they used fresh oil each time. It may be more expensive, but it certainly is healthier. Be careful of most fats, they back up in the body. I believe they may be another big reason why people get sick. (Remember a cold is a cleansing, necessary to keep the body in balance; healthy.) You are what you eat. Remember to read the ingredients label. At least if you cook at home you know what the ingredients label says. You have a better chance of knowing what you're getting.

Unsaturated fat, and polyunsaturated fat, now there's your healthy fats. The following are much better oils to use: Olive oil, sesame oil, sunflower oil, non-GMO corn oil, safflower oil. (It's hard for me to believe that cottonseed oil would be good for you, no matter what.) Unsaturated fats are liquid at room temperature. They can leave the body easier than saturated fat. (I'm not sure about canola oil being good for you.)

My suggestion, eat very little fat. Be careful, as some fats will clog up the body, and all fats are high in calories. Don't overdo it. Eat any oil in small amounts. Oil is fat and fat is high in calories. (Again all fats contain some saturated fat, even though they are called unsaturated fats). If you're going to use oil use mostly unsaturated oil.

Be very careful of salad dressing. Salads are very good for you. They are low in calories and high in nutrition. It's what we ad to the salad that has the calories, lots of calories. We ad cheese and croutons which are usually not so great for you. Then we ad salad dressing; lots of it! Check the nutrition facts label to see how many calories per tablespoon are in that salad dressing. I would guess it's extremely high. You might be using anywhere from 400 to 700 or 800 calories, or believe it or not maybe 1000 calories. That's just in the salad dressing.

Diets Don't Work, Knowledge Does.

****

Cook At Home. Home Cooking Is The Best Cooking.

Nothing can compare to a home cooked meal. It tastes better and it's healthier. Cooking can also be therapeutic, especially if you cook using lots of fresh fruits and vegetables. Real food smells good, and has beautiful colors. Cook with love, because love, believe it or not, goes into the food. If you eat out, which people do more and more, try to eat in a restaurant that uses high quality food. I can tell you that is very hard to find. What a shame; profit is more important than people. I think we've lost our minds. We should be able to have both. (Eating low quality food will eventually make us sick, because it's toxic.)

Fasting

I have juiced off and on for many years. Juicing is excellent for you because it offers high nutrition. You can do a juice fast which will allow the body to mostly rest, and will help the body to cleanse. If you fast for more than 2 to 3 days, like I may have said before, make sure that you consult with a physician that understands fasting. The juice I like to make the most is one with carrots as the base, celery as the second base, using quite a lot of parsley, a little bit of beet, and possibly a small amount of ginger. I like to use a masticating juicer because I believe it does not kill the enzymes. But any juicer is better than none. I have done three kinds of fasts. All three work. I have done a Brown Rice fast, which I think is very good. I have also done a juice fast, and I have also done a lemon and real Maple Syrup fast, which I also think is very good. Again, make sure you do fasting under the supervision of a doctor, or someone who specializes in nutrition and understands fasting.

This is what happens when you fast. After about a day, you can feel the body start to detoxify. You start to burp more, pass gas, and the eyes may get some debris in their corners. You might find that your nose starts to run a little bit. You might find that your skin becomes somewhat oily, especially on your head. Your skin may start to break out a little bit. A lot of toxins go into the bloodstream as the cells start to cleanse. From the bloodstream a lot of those toxins go into the urine or the feces. It is important that you drink plenty of water. It is important to have a decent to good bowel movement every day. You have to get rid of those toxins. The body is now cleansing, beginning to throw off waste, toxins, gunk.

The first day of fasting is difficult because you get hungry. You won't lose weight immediately because the body thinks you're going into survival mode. At certain times you may get tired because toxins are going into the bloodstream. As those toxins move out of the body, you will build more and more energy. I can tell you, that you will start to feel better.

If you change your diet, to eat better, the body will also start to cleanse. While that isn't as quick, the body will gradually throw off toxins and you will definitely feel better. All the methods of throwing off waste, such as through the pores will start to happen.

If you are fasting for more than two days, when you start to eat again, start slowly. Give the body a chance to resume digestion. Maybe start with a little apple juice mixed with water.

Once you realize how wonderful you feel by eating real food, it's pretty hard to go back to the old you.

Read on

Interesting Thoughts

I have learned some interesting things about food, that I would like to talk about. All real food has many benefits. The following are little tips that can be very beneficial.

garlic – blood purifier

shitake mushrooms – blood purifier

burdock – blood purifier, found mostly in Asian stores

peppermint – aids digestion and helps to get rid of gas. Drink peppermint tea two or three times a week.

ginger – is the same as peppermint, is a little stronger, use sparingly radish – helps to deal with a feeling of grease in your stomach. Sometimes for instance, french fries and ice cream can give you that greasy feeling. Too much fat.

pineapple – aids digestion

**Use all the above in small amounts

Some thoughts just jumped into my head that are very disturbing and I felt it was important to talk about them.

One thought is about the school lunch program. What are we thinking about that we would feed our children sub quality food. We expect them to want to go to school, to do well, and we feed them pure junk. How can we expect students to do well in school when we feed them subpar food.

My next thought. My wife just read on the internet that someone she knows just had a stent put in, in the hospital, and they brought breakfast to him the following day. Here's a man who has heart issues, probably pretty much clogged up. This is the breakfast that the hospital gave him; eggs, sausage, and milk. I guess the hospital needs to keep their patients coming back. That's three animal proteins, all at the same time, high in fat. Somebody's nuts!

The following are some tools needed in order to take better care of yourself and those that you love.

Pressure cooker – I prefer stainless steel – I use it for making most grains, beans, and some vegetables, such as collards.

High-speed blender – a high-speed blender can be used to make nut butters, soups, natural frozen desserts, salad dressings and sauces, dips and spreads. You can chop with them, and you can make baby food with them.

Masticating juicer – The reason I use a masticating juicer is because it keeps the enzymes alive since it does not create heat. It also keeps more of the nutrition. I feel that a masticating juicer is much better to restore one's health.

Vegetable cutting knife – wherever you can get stainless steel in any of the tools, that's what you want to use. The vegetable knife makes it much easier to cut fruits and vegetables.

Pots and pans – stainless steel or glass, although nonstick surfaces are being sold, I'm still not sure that these surfaces do not leach into the food.

Air Fryer – this is a relatively new tool that's on the market. Once you get used to it, it definitely helps with cooking good food; low in fat or no fat. If you can find an air fryer that's made with stainless steel inserts, that's what I would buy.

Wood utensils – they are easy to buy in the stores, and I either use them or stainless steel. I do not like to use metal against metal if I'm using stainless steel pots.

You will acquire many other pieces of equipment as time goes on, such as measuring cups, rolling pins and who knows what else. Making real food is fun and it's certainly is wonderful to eat.

Read on – you're almost to the end of the book, a book meant to change your life and the lives of those you love, and know.

To the person reading this book, even if you understand, and agree with all that I am saying, I realize that changing your life is not easy. Revamping your diet, to be a better you, takes time. Even if we want to get better, it's difficult to do. We have to learn. We have to have reinforcement. We have to have someone help us. We have to have a teacher. I've had many teachers to help me change my life. I remember every one of them. They were very important to me, and even though I haven't seen them in many years, I still think of them.

So I've opened up a school called YogaMattAcademy.com. The name Yoga Matt is what one of my best friends has called me for years. All of a sudden it seems to have stuck. I love what I've learned and I love to help people. What I say in this book I can help you achieve. Give YogaMattAcademy.com and me a chance. We will work together to be healthier and happier. Once you learn I hope you will do the same and help other people. (Helping other people will put a smile on your face and a song in your heart too. You may even skip a little.) To everyone young and old you can do so much better. To feel better, to look better, to think better. For those of you that have young children, if you change your lifestyle by having better eating habits, a better exercise program and inspirational knowledge, your children will automatically learn, and when they get older, for the most part this is how they will live out their lives. That will even put a bigger smile on your face. I have seen way to many children that are sick, with problems that they should not have. Please, let me help! At least give me a chance.

YogaMattAcademy.com, check it out

Read on

The body is the greatest machine ever created. Remember, the body can cleanse itself. Remember, the body can heal itself.

Each one of us has to take responsibility for our own life. Our own health and happiness. That word responsibility is extremely important. I can give you every idea of how to get your health back. It will not work unless you take the responsibility to give the body the health and happiness that it deserves.

Remember

Eat good, healthy, food.

Drink plenty of good, clean, healthy water.

Have a good, healthy, bowel movement every day.

Try to stay off products, and medication that stops the body from cleansing, unless absolutely necessary.

Get an excellent book on nutrition. A book that breaks down foods and their nutritional values.

Read books, listen to CDs, watch DVDs of people that really know. Stay away from bad restaurants.

Learn to read the nutritional facts and ingredients label on a can or packaged foods.

Take a tall glass of water, and I'll take a tall glass of water. Let's both drink to your health.

Years ago I read a book. It was one of my first books on health. It said a person should be healthy, they should be able to one day ride their bike up a mountain when their much older and then just keel over and die. In other words, we shouldn't be sick like we are, taking all kinds of medication, for most people, all the way through their lives. To your health, to your happiness, to your well-being.

Nobody can live forever, but while you are alive you are entitled to be healthy and happy!

Remember, the rules of the game.

Thank you for reading,

You're Not Sick You're Clogged

The end, or is it just the beginning?

Check out COUPON at the end of the book.

IMPORTANT

This Book, You're Not Sick, You're Clogged, Helps To Explain The Rules Of The Game. How To Keep, Or Regain Your Health.

It Also Explains The Whys Of So,

So Many Health Problems.

Remember Your Body Is A Machine, From Head To Toe, The Greatest Machine Ever Created. Health Problems, The

Way We Have Them, Should Not Be!

Use This Book Like An Instruction Manual To Help Your Body Run Magnificently.

!You're not sick, your clogged!

Look Better, Lose weight
– Get Healthy – Feel Much Better

<u>Keep going</u>

COUPON COMING UP

As I was completing this book I ran across an interesting story. I was in a supermarket when I saw an older couple wearing medical masks. I stopped them and asked why? They did not want to get the flu so they had the masks on. They would not get the flu shot. This was in December. They were in a catch 22. If they don't cleanse they will get sicker. They didn't want an extreme cleansing such as the flu. They were right. After flu season let your body cleanse naturally. Apply what this book talks about.

This book "You're Not Sick You're Clogged" will absolutely help you!

Read on

About the Author

My real name is Matthew David Goldstein. My friends call me Yoga Matt or Swami Matt. I was a nice kid, and I was somewhat shy. I was not a lover of school, and was an average student. I did love to go to school just to see my friends. I was in a choir at school as I got older. I was fairly good at sports. I took four years of woodshop and got A's and B's. I loved fashion and design and was in the clothing business as a career for about 35 years.

As I look back on my life my biggest strength was trying to piece things together, to figure out why! I would always ask a lot of questions. It's amazing that when you ask a lot of questions you do find people that absolutely know the answers. The people are out there and so are the books. The information is out there, you just have to piece it together. Once I felt satisfied that I came to the right conclusion, I would then test out the information. If it worked, I felt it was important to tell other people.

At approximately the age of 30 years old I started having physical problems. My back was going out. I already was on over-the-counter medication for constant acid indigestion. I used medication to stop my nose from being clogged or constantly running, and I had colds at least twice a year. I had sinus headaches and used lots of aspirin. I had a constant problem with dandruff. I was always constipated. Around 40 years of age I was beginning to get psoriasis around the ears. With the back problems I was having I would've probably needed surgery within a year, but thank God that was not my destiny. I had enough of not feeling well. Because I had an inquisitive mind I wanted to know what the heck was going on. I was young and having all kinds of health issues. I wanted to meet people that actually knew how to deal with these problems so my life would be better.

I started to talk to more and more people as I got older. I wanted to know why and how to get healthy without medication and without surgery. I had a father that had his own health issues. When I was a boy my father started to read a monthly magazine called Reader's Digest. My father was starting to learn. By the time I was in my thirties I started to finally listen to my dad. I call my father the original guru. My father was way ahead of his time. He lived to be three months shy of 100 years old. He didn't live that long because of luck, my father truly worked on it.

I was starting to listen to him as well as other people. I got certified in Yoga, went to seminars, lectures, etc. I became fascinated with what I was learning. I wanted to know more and more on how to keep healthy. It's amazing what I've learned. Because I've learned so much that absolutely works I needed to write this book and the books to follow. You see the knowledge is out there. I worked very hard to search it out, to learn.

I've just recently opened a website called YogaMattAcademy.com. I hope this web site will be completed no later than May 15, 2019.

Now you know the rest of the story.

I hope you enjoyed and learned from book 1, "You're Not Sick Your Clogged". The truth is out there, pass it on. Help as many people as you can.

YOU'RE NOT SICK, YOU ARE WITHOUT A DOUBT DEFINITELY CLOGGED

coupon to follow

READ ON

COUPON

1st Month Just 5.00

REGISTER NOW AND BECOME A MEMBER FOR JUST 20.00 PER MONTH
$120.00 value (1st 50 members just 20.00 per mo.)

Go To Website: **YogaMattAcademy.com**

Use Promo Code: **GRANT** (1st month just 5.00)

FREE COUPON----------FREE COUPON--------FREE COUPON

Become a Member

Go to and JOIN

YogaMattAcademy.com

$120.00 value just 20.00 per mo.

Register now first 50 members

1st mo. Just 5.00 Become a Member

****

LOOK BETTER, FEEL BETTER, THINK BETTER

Use promo code: GRANT

FREE COUPON-------------------------------------FREE COUPON-